This book was compiled by Daniel Melehi
with the A.I assistance of Inventabot

<u>Dedication</u>

I hope this helps all of my wonderful readers achieve all their goals in their business. And I would like to thank my wonderful wife for all of her continued support in all my ventures.

Table of Contents

Chapter 1: The Anatomy of Breathing

Breathing is a natural process of our body that allows us to take in oxygen and release carbon dioxide. But have you ever wondered how this process actually takes place? In this chapter, we will delve deeper into the anatomy of breathing.

THE RESPIRATORY SYSTEM

The respiratory system is responsible for the process of breathing. It consists of the following organs:

Nose and Mouth

The nose and mouth are the entry points of air into the respiratory system. The nose serves as a filter that removes impurities, warms and humidifies the air before it enters the lungs. It also contains tiny hairs called cilia that trap dust and other foreign particles.

Pharynx and Larynx

The pharynx and larynx are the passages that connect the nose and mouth to the trachea. The larynx contains the vocal cords that vibrate to produce sound during speech.

Trachea and Bronchi

The trachea, also known as the windpipe, is a tube-like structure that connects the larynx to the bronchi. It is lined with mucus and cilia that help trap and remove foreign particles. At the base of the trachea, it divides into two bronchi – one leading to each lung.

Lungs

The lungs are the main organs of the respiratory system. They are protected by the ribcage and consist of thousands of tiny air sacs called alveoli where gas exchange occurs. Oxygen from the air is absorbed by the blood in the alveoli, while carbon dioxide produced by the body is released into the alveoli to be exhaled.

THE MECHANICS OF BREATHING

Breathing is controlled by the diaphragm muscle, which separates the chest cavity from the abdominal cavity. When we inhale, the diaphragm contracts and moves downward, creating more space for the lungs to expand. This allows air to flow into the lungs. When we exhale, the diaphragm relaxes and moves upward, decreasing the space in the lungs and pushing air out.

CONCLUSION

The anatomy of breathing is complex and fascinating. Understanding how our respiratory system works can help us better appreciate the importance of taking care of our lungs. In the next chapter, we will discuss the most common respiratory condition – COPD.

Chapter 2: Understanding COPD

COPD, or Chronic Obstructive Pulmonary Disease, is a term used to describe a group of respiratory conditions that cause breathing difficulties. COPD is a progressive disease, meaning that it gets worse over time.

WHAT CAUSES COPD?

COPD is usually caused by long-term exposure to irritating gases or particles, most commonly from cigarette smoke. Tobacco smoke is the leading cause of COPD, but exposure to air pollution, chemicals, and dust can also contribute to the development of the disease. Genetics can also play a role in the development of COPD.

WHAT ARE THE SYMPTOMS OF COPD?

The symptoms of COPD can vary, but typically include coughing, wheezing, shortness of breath, and chest tightness. These symptoms can be mild at first but can become more severe over time, making it difficult to carry out everyday activities such as walking or climbing stairs.

HOW IS COPD DIAGNOSED?

Doctors can diagnose COPD by performing a series of tests, including a lung function test called spirometry. This test measures how much air a person can breathe in and out, as well as how quickly they can exhale. Other tests may include chest X-rays or CT scans to check for any abnormalities in the lungs.

WHAT ARE THE STAGES OF COPD?

COPD is typically classified into four stages, ranging from mild to very severe. The stages are determined by the severity of breathing difficulties and the amount of airflow obstruction. Treatment options and management of COPD will depend on the stage of the disease.

HOW IS COPD TREATED?

While COPD is a progressive and incurable disease, there are treatments available to manage symptoms and slow down the progression of the disease. Treatment options include medications such as bronchodilators and inhaled steroids, oxygen therapy, pulmonary rehabilitation programs, and lifestyle changes such as quitting smoking and avoiding exposure to irritants. In severe cases, surgery or lung transplantation may be necessary.

Conclusion

Understanding COPD is the first step in managing the disease and improving overall quality of life. Treatment options, lifestyle changes, and management strategies are available to help those with COPD live a fulfilling life despite their condition.

Chapter 3: Diagnosis of COPD

COPD, or chronic obstructive pulmonary disease, is a condition that affects millions of people worldwide. However, diagnosing COPD can be a challenge, as its symptoms can often be mistaken for those of other respiratory conditions or simply attributed to aging. Nonetheless, it's important to receive a proper diagnosis in order to begin treatment and better manage your symptoms. Here are some of the ways that COPD is diagnosed:

MEDICAL HISTORY AND PHYSICAL EXAM

Your doctor will likely begin the diagnosis process by taking a detailed medical history and performing a physical exam. During the medical history, your doctor will ask you questions about your symptoms, such as when they first started, how severe they are, and whether they are worse during certain activities or times of day. Your doctor will also ask about any risk factors you may have for COPD, such as a history of smoking or exposure to environmental pollutants. Next, your doctor will perform a physical exam, which may involve listening to your lungs with a stethoscope and measuring your oxygen levels. Your doctor may also ask you to perform a pulmonary function test, which involves breathing into a machine that measures how much air you can exhale and how quickly you can do so.

PULMONARY FUNCTION TESTING

One of the key tests used to diagnose COPD is known as spirometry. This test measures how much air you can exhale forcefully after taking a deep breath. If you have COPD, this test will reveal that you have reduced airflow to your lungs. In addition to spirometry, your doctor may also perform additional pulmonary function tests, such as a lung volume measurement or a gas diffusion test. These tests can help your doctor determine how severe your COPD is and how well your lungs are functioning overall.

IMAGING TESTS

In some cases, your doctor may also order imaging tests to help diagnose COPD. A chest X-ray can help your doctor rule out other respiratory conditions or detect lung damage caused by COPD. A CT scan, on the other hand, can provide more detailed images of your lungs and help your doctor identify potential causes of your symptoms.

ARTERIAL BLOOD GAS TEST

In some cases, your doctor may also order an arterial blood gas test to measure the levels of oxygen and carbon dioxide in your blood. This test can help your doctor determine how well your lungs are functioning and whether additional oxygen therapy may be necessary.

CONCLUSION

COPD can be a challenging condition to diagnose, given its similarities to other respiratory conditions and the fact that its symptoms may be attributed to aging. However, by taking a detailed medical history, performing a physical exam and pulmonary function tests, and ordering imaging and blood tests, your doctor can make an accurate diagnosis and begin treatment to help you better manage your symptoms.

Chapter 4: Treatment Options for COPD

After being diagnosed with COPD, it is essential to work closely with a healthcare provider to develop a comprehensive plan to manage the condition. COPD treatment aims to reduce symptoms, improve lung function, and prevent exacerbations.

1. MEDICATIONS

There are several types of medications available for COPD treatment. Each medication works differently to manage symptoms and improve lung function. The most common medications include bronchodilators and corticosteroids. Bronchodilators work by relaxing the muscles around the airways, making it easier to breathe. These are available in short-acting and long-acting forms. Short-acting bronchodilators provide quick relief of symptoms but are short-lived, while long-acting bronchodilators are taken regularly to prevent symptoms from occurring. Corticosteroids, on the other hand, work by reducing inflammation in the airways. These are usually given in an inhaler form, and they can also be taken orally or through injection in severe cases.

2. OXYGEN THERAPY

In some cases, individuals with COPD may require oxygen therapy to improve oxygen levels in the blood. Oxygen is administered through a nasal cannula or face mask, and it can be used during the day or overnight.

3. PULMONARY REHABILITATION

Pulmonary rehabilitation is a program that allows individuals with COPD to work with a team of healthcare professionals to improve their overall lung function. The program typically includes exercise training, breathing techniques, and nutritional counseling.

4. SURGERY

In severe cases, surgery may be necessary to improve lung function. Lung volume reduction surgery involves removing a portion of damaged lung tissue to help the remaining healthy lung tissue work more efficiently. In some cases, a lung transplant may be an option.

Conclusion

COPD treatment options aim to manage symptoms and improve lung function to help individuals maintain their quality of life. It is crucial to work closely with a healthcare provider to develop a personalized treatment plan that works best for each individual case.

Chapter 5: Medications for COPD

Medications play an essential role in the treatment of COPD. Although there is no cure for the disease, several different types of medications can help individuals manage their symptoms and improve their quality of life. In this chapter, we'll explore the various medications used to treat COPD and discuss how they work.

BRONCHODILATORS

Bronchodilators are a type of medication that relaxes the muscles around the airways, making it easier to breathe. They are available in two categories: short-acting and long-acting bronchodilators. Short-acting bronchodilators are usually taken as needed to relieve sudden symptoms. They work quickly and are effective for up to four to six hours. Examples of short-acting bronchodilators include albuterol (ProAir

HFA, Ventolin HFA, others) and ipratropium (Combivent, DuoNeb). Long-acting bronchodilators, on the other hand, are used to prevent symptoms and are usually taken once or twice daily. These medications can provide relief for up to 12-24 hours. Some examples include tiotropium (Spiriva), formoterol (Foradil, Perforomist), and salmeterol (Serevent).

INHALED CORTICOSTEROIDS

In addition to bronchodilators, inhaled corticosteroids may also be prescribed to prevent worsening of COPD symptoms. These medications work by reducing inflammation in the airways. Examples include fluticasone (Flovent HFA), budesonide (Pulmicort Flexhaler), and mometasone (Asmanex HFA). It's important to note that these medications are usually used in combination with long-acting bronchodilators. Additionally, long-term use of inhaled corticosteroids can increase the risk of side effects such as osteoporosis, cataracts, and adrenal insufficiency. Regular monitoring is required to identify and manage any potential side effects.

COMBINATION MEDICATIONS

Combination medications, as their name suggests, are a blend of bronchodilators and corticosteroids. These medications can provide relief for patients who have COPD symptoms that are not well-controlled by bronchodilators alone. Examples include Advair Diskus (fluticasone and salmeterol), Symbicort (budesonide and formoterol), and Breo Ellipta (fluticasone and vilanterol).

PHOSPHODIESTERASE-4 INHIBITORS

Phosphodiesterase-4 (PDE4) inhibitors are a type of medication that reduces the inflammation in the lungs, which can help to relieve COPD symptoms. Roflumilast (Daliresp) is an example of a PDE4 inhibitor that is often prescribed to treat COPD. This medication can cause side effects such as weight loss, upset stomach, and mood changes.

ANTIBIOTICS AND VACCINATIONS

Antibiotics and vaccinations are also important in the management of COPD. Antibiotics are used to treat bacterial infections that can cause exacerbations, which can worsen COPD symptoms. Vaccinations such as influenza vaccines and pneumococcal vaccines can help to prevent infections in the first place.

Conclusion

Medications are an essential component in the management of COPD. Different types of medications may be used alone or in combination to help control symptoms and improve quality of life for individuals with COPD. It's important to work closely with a healthcare provider to identify the right medications and dosages for each patient. Additionally, regular monitoring is required to manage any potential side effects and ensure that the medications remain effective.

Chapter 6: Oxygen Therapy

THE IMPORTANCE OF OXYGEN THERAPY

Oxygen is crucial for our bodies to function properly. When you have COPD or another respiratory condition that affects your ability to breathe, it can be difficult to get the amount of oxygen you need. This is where oxygen therapy comes in. Oxygen therapy involves using a machine to deliver oxygen to your lungs, either through a mask or nasal prongs.

Who Needs Oxygen Therapy?

Not everyone with COPD needs oxygen therapy, but it can be very helpful for those with more advanced stage COPD. Your doctor may recommend oxygen therapy if your blood oxygen levels are consistently low, even with other treatments.

Types of Oxygen Therapy

There are a few different types of oxygen therapy available: - **Compressed oxygen:** This involves using tanks of compressed oxygen to deliver oxygen through a mask or nasal prongs. - **Liquid oxygen:** This involves using a machine to convert liquid oxygen into a gas, which can then be delivered through a mask or nasal prongs. - **Oxygen concentrators:** This is a machine that pulls oxygen from the air and delivers it through a mask or nasal prongs. Your doctor can help you determine which type of oxygen therapy is best for you.

Using Oxygen Therapy at Home

If you've been prescribed oxygen therapy, you'll likely need to use it at home. It's important to follow your doctor's instructions carefully to ensure you're using the machine properly and getting the correct amount of oxygen.

Traveling with Oxygen Therapy

If you need to travel with your oxygen machine, there are a few things to consider. You'll need to arrange for oxygen delivery at your destination, and you'll also need to make sure your machine is portable and easy to transport.

Potential Side Effects

While oxygen therapy can be very helpful, there are some potential side effects to keep in mind. These can include dry nose or mouth, nosebleeds, and skin irritation from the mask or prongs. Talk to your doctor if you experience any of these side effects.

Chapter 7: Lifestyle Changes for Managing COPD

Living with COPD can be challenging, but there are several lifestyle changes you can make that may help manage the symptoms and improve your quality of life. Making certain adjustments in your daily routine can go a long way in managing COPD. Here are some lifestyle changes that may help you:

QUIT SMOKING

Smoking is one of the leading causes of COPD, therefore, quitting smoking is the most important thing you can do to manage your symptoms. Quitting may be hard, but there are several resources available that can help you quit smoking for good. Consulting a doctor, taking nicotine replacement therapy, and seeking support from family and friends can greatly improve your chances of successfully quitting smoking.

PREVENT RESPIRATORY INFECTIONS

COPD patients are more vulnerable to respiratory infections, which can significantly exacerbate their condition. Taking preventative measures such as washing your hands frequently, getting vaccinated for flu and pneumonia, and avoiding close contact with sick people can help prevent respiratory infections.

EAT A BALANCED DIET

Maintaining a balanced diet is crucial for managing COPD. Consuming a variety of nutrient-rich foods such as fruits, vegetables, lean proteins, and whole grains may help improve lung function and overall health.

EXERCISE REGULARLY

Although exercise may seem daunting for COPD patients, it can actually help improve lung function, boost energy levels, and improve overall fitness. Engaging in low-impact exercises such as walking, swimming, and cycling may help improve your breathing and overall health.

AVOID EXTREME TEMPERATURES

Extreme temperatures can be overwhelming for COPD patients, especially extreme cold. Therefore, it is important to avoid spending prolonged periods of time in extreme weather conditions that may aggravate your COPD symptoms.

REDUCE STRESS

Stress can exacerbate COPD symptoms, thus it is important to find ways to manage stress levels. Participating in relaxation activities such as deep breathing, yoga, or massage therapy may help reduce stress levels and improve overall wellness. By incorporating these lifestyle changes into your daily routine, you may be able to manage your COPD symptoms more effectively and improve your overall quality of life.

Chapter 8: Managing COPD Exacerbations

COPD exacerbations are acute episodes of symptom worsening that can cause significant complications and even lead to hospitalization. Managing COPD exacerbations is crucial to maintain a patient's quality of life.

COPD EXACERBATION TRIGGERS

Exacerbations can be triggered by a variety of factors, including viral or bacterial infections, environmental pollution, and changes in weather. It is important to identify triggers and avoid them as much as possible to prevent exacerbations.

RECOGNIZING EXACERBATION SYMPTOMS

The symptoms of COPD exacerbation can vary from patient to patient, but common symptoms include shortness of breath, coughing, wheezing, chest tightness, and increased production of mucus. Patients with COPD should be aware of these symptoms and take action as soon as possible if they begin to experience any of them.

MANAGING EXACERBATIONS

The management of COPD exacerbations involves a combined effort of the patient and healthcare provider. The first step in managing an exacerbation is to increase medication usage as prescribed, including the quick-relief medications. Oxygen therapy may also be necessary. It is important to rest and avoid any strenuous physical activity during exacerbations. Drinking plenty of fluids is also essential in order to prevent dehydration. Patients should also be educated on the importance of having an action plan in place in case of exacerbations. An action plan can help patients and their caregivers recognize the early warning signs of an exacerbation and take appropriate steps to manage it, such as increasing medication and contacting healthcare providers for advice.

WHEN TO SEEK MEDICAL HELP

In some cases, managing a COPD exacerbation at home may not be enough, and medical attention may be necessary. Patients should seek medical help immediately if they experience severe symptoms such as blue lips or fingernails, confusion, difficulty speaking, or extreme shortness of breath.

CONCLUSION

Managing COPD exacerbations is an essential part of COPD management. Patients should be aware of the triggers and symptoms of exacerbations and have an action plan in place to manage them. Working closely with healthcare providers can also help patients achieve the best possible outcomes in managing COPD exacerbations.

Chapter 9: The Importance of Exercise in COPD

Living with COPD can significantly impact a person's ability to perform everyday tasks with ease. Physical exertion can cause shortness of breath, fatigue, and overall weakness. However, despite these challenges, it's essential for individuals diagnosed with COPD to engage in exercise as part of their treatment plan.

UNDERSTANDING THE BENEFITS OF EXERCISE

Although it may seem counterintuitive to exert oneself while battling a condition that causes shortness of breath and fatigue, exercise has numerous benefits for individuals with COPD. Regular physical activity can improve overall fitness, increase lung capacity, and decrease the risk of developing other health complications commonly associated with COPD. One of the most significant benefits of exercise for those with COPD is an increase in stamina. Over time, engaging in physical activity can help the body use oxygen more efficiently, leading to an overall improvement in endurance. Regular exercise can also help individuals with COPD maintain a healthy weight, reducing the risk of additional health complications such as heart disease, diabetes, and joint problems.

TYPES OF EXERCISE FOR INDIVIDUALS WITH COPD

It's crucial for individuals with COPD to engage in physical activity that is safe, effective, and takes their specific needs into account. While vigorous activity is generally not recommended, there are several types of exercise that are safe and commonly prescribed as part of a COPD treatment plan. Low-impact exercises such as walking, cycling, and swimming are ideal for individuals with COPD as they put minimal strain on the respiratory system.

Strength training exercises can also be beneficial, helping to increase muscle mass and further improve overall fitness.

IMPORTANT CONSIDERATIONS

Before starting any exercise routine, it's essential for individuals with COPD to consult with their doctor or a qualified healthcare professional. They can help determine the right type and intensity of exercise and provide guidance on how to safely and effectively incorporate physical activity into a daily routine. It's also important to monitor any physical changes that may occur while engaging in exercise, such as shortness of breath or chest pain. This information can help healthcare professionals modify an individual's exercise routine to better suit their specific needs and abilities.

Conclusion

Engaging in regular exercise is vital for individuals with COPD. While it may seem daunting at first, understanding the benefits of physical activity and working with healthcare professionals to establish a safe and effective routine can lead to significant improvements in overall health and quality of life.

Chapter 10: Nutrition and COPD

COPD can cause a range of symptoms that can make eating a challenge. Feeling short of breath, coughing, and wheezing may make it difficult to eat enough food to maintain a healthy weight. However, good nutrition plays a key role in managing COPD symptoms, preventing infections, and reducing flare-ups.

UNDERSTANDING NUTRITIONAL NEEDS FOR COPD PATIENTS

COPD patients have unique nutritional needs due to the extra energy expenditure used in breathing and maintaining physical activity, as well as the increased risk of malnutrition. The condition can cause a loss of appetite, which can make it hard to eat enough. It's important to eat nutrient-dense foods to optimize energy intake. COPD patients should aim to consume enough vitamins, minerals, and protein to promote lung health, muscle function and overall wellbeing.

CHOOSING FOODS FOR COPD PATIENTS

Fruits and vegetables are essential sources of vitamins, minerals, and antioxidants that help protect the lungs. Dark, leafy greens, berries, citrus fruit, and sweet potatoes are especially good choices for COPD patients. Foods high in protein, such as lean meats, poultry, fish, dairy, eggs and legumes can help rebuild and maintain muscle mass. This is particularly important in advanced stages of COPD where muscle wasting can have harmful effects on respiratory function. Avoiding processed and fast foods which are high in saturated and trans fats, and instead opting for healthy fats like olive oil, nuts, and seeds, can help decrease inflammation and improve lung function.

MANAGING WEIGHT AND FLUID INTAKE

COPD can cause weight gain or loss. Some people with COPD are overweight due to a sedentary lifestyle and inactivity, while others may be underweight from a loss of appetite or malabsorption of nutrients. Maintaining a healthy weight is important to reduce pressure on the lungs, improve breathing and energy levels. Drinking plenty of fluids, especially water, helps keep mucus thin and easy to cough up, which can reduce airway inflammation associated with COPD.

WORKING WITH A DIETITIAN

Working with a registered dietitian can be helpful for COPD patients to develop a nutrition plan tailored to their specific needs. A dietitian can assist patients in planning meals, controlling portion sizes, and avoiding foods that may trigger COPD symptoms, such as bloating, gas, or heartburn. Dietary supplements can also be prescribed if needed.

Conclusion

As nutrition plays a crucial role in COPD management, a balanced and nutrient-dense diet is important for patients with COPD. Eating a balanced diet rich in fruits, vegetables, lean protein, and healthy fats along with drinking enough fluids can help improve lung function, energy levels, and quality of life.

Chapter 11: Alternative Therapies for COPD

When it comes to managing COPD, traditional treatments such as medication, oxygen therapy, and lifestyle changes are often the primary focus. However, many individuals with COPD also turn to alternative therapies to help alleviate symptoms and improve their overall quality of life.

ACUPUNCTURE

Acupuncture is a traditional Chinese medicine practice that involves inserting thin needles into specific points on the body to alleviate pain and promote healing. For individuals with COPD, acupuncture may help to reduce inflammation, relieve chest tightness and shortness of breath, and improve overall breathing function. While research on the effectiveness of acupuncture in treating COPD is limited, some studies have shown promising results, particularly in reducing breathlessness and improving exercise capacity. It's important to note that acupuncture should only be performed by a licensed and trained acupuncturist to minimize the risk of complications.

HERBAL MEDICINE

Herbal medicine is another alternative therapy used by some individuals with COPD to help manage symptoms. Specifically, certain herbs such as licorice root, ginseng, and eucalyptus have been found to have anti-inflammatory properties and may help to reduce inflammation in the airways, making breathing easier. However, it's important to note that herbal medicine can have potentially harmful interactions with medications and may not be safe for everyone, particularly those with liver or kidney problems. Before trying any herbal remedies, it's important to consult with a healthcare provider and a licensed herbalist to ensure safety and effectiveness.

MEDITATION

Meditation is a mind-body practice that involves focusing attention and relaxing the body to reduce stress and promote overall well-being. For individuals with COPD, meditation may help to reduce anxiety, improve breathing function, and promote relaxation. Several studies have suggested that regular meditation practice may lead to improvements in breathing function and quality of life in individuals with COPD. Meditation can be done in various forms, including guided meditation, mindfulness meditation, and yoga. It's important to find a style of meditation that works best for you and to practice regularly for optimal benefit.

CONCLUSION

While alternative therapies may not be the primary treatment for COPD, they can provide additional support and symptom management for individuals with this chronic respiratory condition. It's important to discuss any alternative therapies with a healthcare provider before trying them and to use them in conjunction with traditional treatments for optimal benefit.

Chapter 12: COPD and Mental Health

Living with COPD can be challenging and stressful. COPD and other respiratory conditions can often lead to feelings of anxiety, depression, and other mental health concerns. In this chapter, we will discuss the connection between COPD and mental health, as well as some coping strategies that can help improve overall well-being.

THE LINK BETWEEN COPD AND MENTAL HEALTH

The impact of COPD on mental health cannot be overstated. COPD can be difficult to manage, with patients experiencing breathing difficulties, fatigue, and chronic pain. This can lead to feelings of isolation, frustration, and anxiety. In some cases, COPD can also contribute to depression, PTSD, and other mental health disorders.

Depression and COPD

Depression is one of the most common mental health concerns among COPD patients. Depression can make it difficult for patients to follow their treatment plan, and can worsen COPD symptoms. In some cases, depression can also increase the risk of hospitalization and reduce overall quality of life. If you are experiencing symptoms of depression such as feeling sad or hopeless, losing interest in activities you once enjoyed, or having trouble sleeping, it's important to talk to your healthcare provider. There are several treatment options available for depression, including antidepressant medications, talk therapy, and lifestyle changes.

Anxiety and COPD

Anxiety is another common mental health concern among COPD patients. Anxiety can lead to shortness of breath, muscle tension, and a rapid heartbeat, which can exacerbate COPD symptoms. In some cases, anxiety can also contribute to panic attacks, social isolation, and other mental health concerns. If you are experiencing symptoms of anxiety such as feeling nervous or tense, having trouble sleeping, or experiencing panic attacks, it's important to talk to your healthcare provider. There are several treatment options available for anxiety, including anti-anxiety medications, talk therapy, and stress-reduction techniques like meditation and deep breathing exercises.

COPING STRATEGIES FOR IMPROVED MENTAL HEALTH

There are several coping strategies that can help improve mental health and overall well-being for COPD patients.

Support Groups

Joining a support group can help COPD patients feel less isolated and more connected to others who are facing similar challenges. Support groups can provide opportunities for socializing, sharing coping strategies, and learning about new treatment options.

Exercise

Exercise can help improve physical and mental health for COPD patients. Exercise can help improve lung function, reduce stress, and boost overall well-being. Talk to your healthcare provider about safe exercise options for COPD patients, including pulmonary rehabilitation programs and low-impact activities like walking or swimming.

Relaxation Techniques

Practicing relaxation techniques like meditation, deep breathing exercises, or yoga can help reduce stress and improve overall mental health. These techniques can help COPD patients feel less anxious and more relaxed, which can improve breathing and reduce symptoms.

CONCLUSION

COPD and other respiratory conditions can have a significant impact on mental health and well-being. It's important for COPD patients to prioritize their mental health and wellbeing, and to seek treatment and support as needed. With the right care and coping strategies, it is possible to manage COPD and improve quality of life.

Chapter 13: Coping Strategies for Anxiety and Depression

Living with COPD and respiratory conditions can be challenging, and for many people, it can lead to feelings of anxiety and depression. Coping with these emotions is an important part of managing your condition. Here are some strategies that can help:

IDENTIFY YOUR TRIGGERS

One of the first steps to coping with anxiety and depression is to identify what triggers these emotions. Do you feel more anxious when you are short of breath? Are there certain activities or situations that make you feel depressed? Once you identify your triggers, it becomes easier to manage your emotions.

EXERCISE REGULARLY

Exercise is a great way to improve your mood and manage anxiety and depression. Even gentle exercises like yoga or walking can help to reduce stress and improve your mental health. Check with your doctor before starting a new exercise program.

PRACTICE RELAXATION TECHNIQUES

Relaxation techniques like deep breathing, meditation, and progressive muscle relaxation can all help to reduce stress and anxiety. These practices can be done anywhere and at any time, so they are an effective way to manage your emotions on the go.

SEEK SUPPORT

It's important to have a support network when dealing with anxiety and depression. This can include friends, family members, or a mental health professional. Talking about your emotions with someone you trust can help to reduce stress and provide perspective on your situation.

FIND JOY IN EVERYDAY ACTIVITIES

Depression can make it difficult to find joy in everyday activities. However, it's important to make an effort to engage in things that bring you pleasure, whether it's reading a book, watching a movie, or spending time with friends. These small moments of happiness can add up over time and improve your overall well-being.

TAKE CARE OF YOURSELF

Self-care is an important part of managing anxiety and depression. This includes getting enough rest, eating a healthy diet, and practicing good hygiene. Taking care of your physical health can also improve your mental health.

Conclusion

Coping with anxiety and depression is a process, and it's important to be patient and compassionate with yourself. By identifying your triggers, staying active, seeking support, and practicing self-care, you can better manage your emotions and improve your overall quality of life.

Chapter 14: Traveling with COPD

For COPD patients, traveling can often be a daunting experience, and it's important to plan ahead to ensure that your trip is safe and enjoyable. Here are some tips to help make your travels smoother:

CONSULT WITH YOUR DOCTOR BEFORE YOU TRAVEL

Before your trip, it's essential to consult with your doctor to make sure that traveling is safe for you. Your doctor can help you determine if there are any precautions you need to take or vaccines you should receive before you travel.

PLAN AHEAD

When traveling with COPD, it's important to plan your trip well in advance. This will give you time to make any necessary accommodations, such as booking a hotel room with a non-smoking policy or arranging for oxygen at your destination.

CONSIDER YOUR MODE OF TRANSPORTATION

When choosing a mode of transportation, consider how it will affect your breathing. For example, if you're traveling by air, make sure to book a non-stop flight to reduce the number of times you need to navigate your way through an airport or wait in a crowded terminal. If you're traveling by car, plan frequent breaks to get out and stretch your legs.

PREPARE YOUR MEDICATIONS AND OXYGEN

Make sure to pack enough medication for your entire trip, as well as an extra supply in case of any unexpected delays. If you require oxygen, arrange for it to be available at your destination and make sure to bring extra oxygen tanks with you on your trip.

STAY HYDRATED

Dehydration can worsen COPD symptoms, so it's important to drink plenty of fluids during your travels. Make sure to bring a reusable water bottle with you and refill it throughout your trip.

TAKE IT SLOW

Traveling can be exhausting for anyone, but it can be especially taxing for those with COPD. Take your time and don't push yourself too hard. Plan for regular breaks to rest and catch your breath, and try not to overexert yourself while on vacation.

CONCLUSION

Traveling with COPD can be challenging, but with the right preparation, it can also be a rewarding and enjoyable experience. By planning ahead, consulting with your doctor, and taking the necessary precautions, you can help ensure that your trip is safe and comfortable.

Remember, don't let your COPD hold you back from exploring the world and creating new memories!

Chapter 15: Living with COPD: Advice from Patients

Living with COPD can be challenging, but you're not alone. Many patients have learned how to manage their symptoms and live a fulfilling life. In this chapter, we will share some advice from patients who have been living with COPD.

JOIN A SUPPORT GROUP

One of the most important things you can do is to join a support group. You can find them online or in-person. A support group will connect you with others who are dealing with the same challenges. You will be able to share your experiences and learn from others. You may also find that being part of a group will give you some sense of purpose.

EXERCISE REGULARLY

Exercise is an important part of managing COPD. You should aim to do some type of exercise every day, even if it's just a short walk. Exercise will help to improve your lung function and make it easier for you to breathe. It will also help you maintain a healthy weight, which is important for managing COPD.

CONSIDER PULMONARY REHABILITATION

Pulmonary rehabilitation is a program that is designed to help patients with COPD improve their quality of life. It involves working with a team of healthcare professionals to develop an individualized treatment plan. The plan may include exercise, breathing techniques, and education about COPD. Talk to your doctor about whether pulmonary rehabilitation may be right for you.

LEARN TO MANAGE STRESS

Stress can worsen COPD symptoms, so it's important to find ways to manage stress. You may want to try meditation or deep breathing exercises. You may also find it helpful to talk to a mental health professional.

AVOID TRIGGERS

Certain things can trigger COPD symptoms, such as cigarette smoke, air pollution, and allergens. It's important to identify your triggers and try to avoid them as much as possible. If you do come into contact with a trigger, try to remove yourself from the situation as quickly as possible.

COMMUNICATE WITH YOUR HEALTHCARE TEAM

Your healthcare team is there to help you manage your COPD. It's important to communicate openly and honestly with them. Tell your doctor about any changes in your symptoms or any new symptoms you may be experiencing. They may be able to adjust your treatment plan to better manage your symptoms.

TAKE CARE OF YOUR MENTAL HEALTH

Living with COPD can be stressful and overwhelming. It's important to take care of your mental health by seeking support when needed and taking steps to manage stress. You may also want to consider talking to a mental health professional if you are experiencing anxiety or depression.

Conclusion

Living with COPD can present many challenges, but it's important to remember that you're not alone. By joining a support group, exercising regularly, considering pulmonary rehabilitation, managing stress, avoiding triggers, communicating with your healthcare team, and taking care of your mental health, you can effectively manage your COPD and lead a fulfilling life.

Chapter 16: Understanding Other Respiratory Conditions

When it comes to respiratory conditions, there are many different types beyond just chronic obstructive pulmonary disease (COPD). While COPD is the fourth leading cause of death worldwide, these other conditions can also be serious and require proper treatment and management. Here are some of the most common respiratory conditions:

ASTHMA

Asthma is a chronic condition that affects the airways and makes it difficult to breathe. It can cause wheezing, shortness of breath, chest tightness, and coughing. Asthma attacks can be triggered by a variety of factors, including allergens, exercise, and stress. Treatment for asthma may involve medication such as inhalers, as well as lifestyle changes to avoid triggers.

BRONCHITIS

Bronchitis is an inflammation of the bronchial tubes, which are the airways that lead to the lungs. It can be acute or chronic, with acute bronchitis usually caused by a virus and chronic bronchitis often linked to smoking. Symptoms of bronchitis include coughing, chest discomfort, and difficulty breathing. Treatment may involve medication, such as bronchodilators, as well as rest and hydration.

CYSTIC FIBROSIS

Cystic fibrosis is a genetic condition that affects the respiratory, digestive, and reproductive systems. It causes a buildup of thick, sticky mucus that clogs the airways and makes it difficult to breathe. Treatment for cystic fibrosis may involve medication, such as antibiotics or mucus-thinning drugs, as well as airway clearance techniques and exercise.

EMPHYSEMA

Emphysema is a type of COPD that specifically affects the air sacs in the lungs. It causes these sacs to lose their elasticity, which makes it difficult to exhale and get rid of air. Symptoms of emphysema include coughing, wheezing, and shortness of breath. Treatment may involve medication, oxygen therapy, and lifestyle changes such as quitting smoking.

PNEUMONIA

Pneumonia is an infection of the lungs that can be caused by bacteria, viruses, or fungi. Symptoms may include coughing, fever, and difficulty breathing. Treatment for pneumonia may involve antibiotics, antiviral medication, or antifungal medication, depending on the underlying cause.

TUBERCULOSIS

Tuberculosis (TB) is a bacterial infection that primarily affects the lungs. It is spread through the air when an infected person coughs or sneezes. Symptoms of TB may include coughing, chest pain, and fever.

Treatment typically involves a combination of medications over several months.

LUNG CANCER

Lung cancer is a type of cancer that begins in the lungs. It is often linked to smoking, but can also be caused by exposure to other harmful substances. Symptoms may include coughing, chest discomfort, and shortness of breath. Treatment for lung cancer may involve surgery, chemotherapy, radiation, or a combination of these approaches. In conclusion, while COPD is a serious respiratory condition, there are many other types of conditions that can affect the lungs. It is important to understand the symptoms and treatment options for these conditions in order to manage respiratory health effectively.

Chapter 17: Asthma and COPD: What's the Difference?

THE BASICS OF ASTHMA AND COPD

Asthma and chronic obstructive pulmonary disease (COPD) are both respiratory disorders that can cause breathing difficulties. People with asthma experience inflammation and narrowing of the airways, which can cause wheezing, coughing, and shortness of breath. COPD, on the other hand, is a chronic and progressive disease that results in increasing airflow obstruction and difficulty in breathing. Although asthma and COPD share some similar symptoms, they are different conditions with unique causes and treatments.

CAUSES AND TRIGGERS OF ASTHMA

Asthma is caused by a combination of genetic and environmental factors. Common triggers for asthma symptoms include allergens such as dust mites, pollen, and animal dander, air pollution, respiratory infections, exercise, and stress. Inflammation of the airways makes them more sensitive to these triggers and causes symptoms to flare up.

CAUSES AND TRIGGERS OF COPD

COPD is most commonly caused by smoking, although exposure to air pollution, chemical fumes, and dust can also contribute to the development of the disease. The primary symptom of COPD is breathlessness, which is caused by progressive lung damage. This results in narrowing of the airways and destruction of lung tissue over time.

SYMPTOMS OF ASTHMA AND COPD

The symptoms of asthma and COPD can overlap, but there are some differences. In patients with asthma, symptoms can be intermittent and may not be present all the time. Symptoms can include wheezing, coughing, shortness of breath, and chest tightness. In contrast, COPD symptoms are usually persistent and worsen over time. These symptoms include coughing, excessive mucus production, and shortness of breath, which can limit physical activity.

TREATMENTS FOR ASTHMA AND COPD

Treatment options for asthma include inhaled corticosteroids and bronchodilators, which help to reduce inflammation and open the airways. Asthma can also be managed by avoiding triggers and improving overall health through lifestyle changes like quitting smoking and maintaining a healthy weight. COPD treatments include bronchodilators and inhaled corticosteroids, as well as oxygen therapy in more severe cases. Pulmonary rehabilitation and regular exercise are also important in improving lung function and overall quality of life.

CONCLUSION

Although asthma and COPD have some similarities, they are distinct respiratory diseases with different causes, symptoms, and treatments. If you experience chronic breathing difficulties, it's important to seek medical attention to receive an accurate diagnosis and appropriate treatment. With proper care, people with asthma and COPD can manage their symptoms and enjoy a good quality of life.

Chapter 18: Bronchitis: Acute and Chronic

Bronchitis is a respiratory condition that arises when the bronchial tubes become inflamed and irritated. It is characterized by coughing, chest discomfort, and the production of phlegm. There are two primary types of bronchitis - acute and chronic.

ACUTE BRONCHITIS

Acute bronchitis is the most common form of bronchitis, and it usually develops after a viral infection, such as a cold or flu. This type of bronchitis typically goes away on its own within 1-2 weeks, and symptoms may include:

Symptoms

- Coughing (with or without mucus) - Chest discomfort - Fatigue - Sore throat - Runny/stuffy nose - Body aches

Treatment

If you have acute bronchitis, treatment may include: - Resting - Drinking plenty of fluids - Taking over-the-counter pain/fever reducers - Using a humidifier or taking a hot shower to help ease congestion - Using an inhaler or medication prescribed by your doctor to help open up airways

CHRONIC BRONCHITIS

Chronic bronchitis is a more serious form of bronchitis that requires ongoing medical attention. It is defined as a productive cough that lasts for at least three months out of the year for two consecutive years. Chronic bronchitis is often caused by smoking and can lead to complications such as:

Symptoms

- Shortness of breath - Chronic cough (with or without mucus) - Wheezing - Fatigue - Chest discomfort - Recurrent respiratory infections

Treatment

If you have chronic bronchitis, treatment may include: - Quitting smoking - Taking medications such as bronchodilators, inhaled corticosteroids, or antibiotics - Using oxygen therapy - Pulmonary rehabilitation (breathing and exercise programs) - Surgery (in rare cases)

Prevention

Since chronic bronchitis is often caused by smoking, the best way to prevent it is to not smoke or quit smoking. Avoiding exposure to lung irritants (such as dust, fumes, and pollution) can also help prevent chronic bronchitis.

Conclusion

Bronchitis can be a serious respiratory condition, and it's important to understand the differences between acute and chronic bronchitis. If you experience symptoms of bronchitis, such as coughing, chest discomfort, or shortness of breath, see your doctor right away. With proper diagnosis and treatment, most people with bronchitis can manage their symptoms and live a healthy life.

Chapter 19: Cystic Fibrosis: A Genetic Respiratory Condition

Cystic fibrosis (CF) is a genetic respiratory disease that causes severe damage to the lungs, digestive system, and other organs in the body. CF is caused by a mutation in the cystic fibrosis transmembrane conductance regulator (CFTR) gene, which produces a protein that is responsible for regulating the balance of salt and water in the body's cells.

SYMPTOMS OF CYSTIC FIBROSIS

CF is a progressive disease that can affect different parts of the body in different ways. The symptoms of CF can vary widely from person to person, but some common symptoms include:

- Difficulty breathing, wheezing, and coughing
- Thick mucus that clogs the airways and makes it hard to breathe
- Frequent lung infections, such as pneumonia or bronchitis
- Poor growth or weight gain, despite a healthy appetite
- Coughing up blood
- Clubbing of the fingers and toes
- Frequent sinus infections
- Constipation or diarrhea
- Pancreatic insufficiency, which can lead to malnutrition and diabetes
- Infertility in males, due to the absence of the vas deferens

DIAGNOSIS OF CYSTIC FIBROSIS

CF is usually diagnosed in infancy or early childhood through a blood test or a sweat test, which measures the level of salt in the sweat. Genetic testing can also be used to identify the mutation in the CFTR gene.

TREATMENT OF CYSTIC FIBROSIS

While there is no cure for CF, there are a number of treatment options available that can help manage the symptoms of the disease, including:

- Antibiotics to treat lung infections
- Bronchodilators to help open up the airways
- Mucus thinning medications to make it easier to cough up mucus
- Chest physical therapy, which involves using a series of techniques to loosen and remove mucus from the lungs
- Nutritional supplements and a high-calorie diet to support growth and weight gain
- Enzyme replacement therapy to improve digestion and nutrient absorption
- Lung transplant for those with severe lung damage

COPING WITH CYSTIC FIBROSIS

Living with CF can be challenging, but there are many resources available to help patients and their families cope with the disease. This may include support groups, counseling, and education about the disease and its treatments. It is important for people with CF to maintain a healthy lifestyle, including regular exercise and a nutritious diet. They should also take steps to protect themselves from infections, such as washing their hands frequently and avoiding large crowds during cold and flu season.

The Future of Cystic Fibrosis Research

Researchers are constantly working to develop new treatments and therapies for CF. Some of the most promising areas of research include:

- Gene therapy to replace or correct the mutated CFTR gene
- Drugs that target specific mutations in the CFTR gene
- Stem cell therapy to repair damaged lung tissue

With ongoing research and advancements in treatment, there is hope for a better future for people with cystic fibrosis.

Chapter 20: Emphysema: A COPD Subtype

Emphysema is a subtype of Chronic Obstructive Pulmonary Disease (COPD) that affects millions of people worldwide. It is a long-term, progressive disease that slowly damages the air sacs, or alveoli, in the lungs, making it difficult to breathe.

WHAT IS EMPHYSEMA?

Emphysema is a condition that affects the lungs. Normally, air moves in and out of the lungs through a series of small airways.

These airways then lead to tiny air sacs called alveoli. When a person has emphysema, the walls between the alveoli are destroyed, causing the air sacs to become larger. This reduces the amount of surface area for gas exchange and can result in breathlessness, coughing, and other respiratory symptoms.

CAUSES OF EMPHYSEMA

The primary cause of emphysema is exposure to cigarette smoke. Other causes of emphysema include long-term exposure to air pollution, secondhand smoke, and occupational exposure to dust and chemicals. Genetics also play a role in the development of emphysema, with some people being more susceptible to the disease than others.

SYMPTOMS OF EMPHYSEMA

The symptoms of emphysema include shortness of breath, wheezing, chest tightness, chronic cough, fatigue, and weight loss. These symptoms can worsen over time, making it difficult to perform daily activities and reducing the overall quality of life.

TREATMENT OF EMPHYSEMA

There is no cure for emphysema, but treatments can help manage symptoms and slow the progression of the disease. Treatment options include medications, oxygen therapy, pulmonary rehabilitation, and surgery in severe cases.

LIFESTYLE CHANGES FOR MANAGING EMPHYSEMA

There are several lifestyle changes that can help manage emphysema symptoms. These include quitting smoking, avoiding air pollution, eating a healthy diet, staying active, and avoiding respiratory infections.

CONCLUSION

Emphysema is a subtype of COPD that affects millions of people worldwide. It is a chronic disease that slowly damages the air sacs in the lungs, making it difficult to breathe. While there is no cure for emphysema, treatment options and lifestyle changes can help manage symptoms and slow the progression of the disease. If you suspect you may have emphysema, speak with your healthcare provider for proper diagnosis and treatment options.

Chapter 21: Pneumonia: Symptoms, Diagnosis, and Treatment

Pneumonia is a respiratory infection that affects the lungs. It can be caused by bacteria, viruses, or fungi. Pneumonia can be serious, especially for older adults, young children, and people with weakened immune systems. In this chapter, we will discuss the symptoms, diagnosis, and treatment of pneumonia.

SYMPTOMS OF PNEUMONIA

The symptoms of pneumonia can vary from person to person. Common symptoms include: - Cough - Fever - Shortness of breath - Chest pain - Fatigue - Sweating - Headaches - Muscle aches If you experience any of these symptoms, it is important to see a doctor as soon as possible. Pneumonia can worsen quickly, especially in high-risk individuals.

DIAGNOSIS OF PNEUMONIA

If you have symptoms of pneumonia, your doctor will likely perform a physical exam and order tests to confirm the diagnosis. Tests may include: - Chest X-ray: A chest X-ray can show signs of pneumonia in the lungs. - Blood tests: Blood tests can detect signs of infection in the body. - Sputum test: This test can help identify the type of bacteria causing the infection.

TREATMENT OF PNEUMONIA

Treatment for pneumonia depends on the cause of the infection. If the infection is bacterial, antibiotics can be prescribed. If the infection is viral, treatment may include rest and over-the-counter medications to manage symptoms. Other treatments may include: - Oxygen therapy: If you are having trouble breathing, oxygen therapy can improve your oxygen levels. - Intravenous fluids: If you are dehydrated due to fever or difficulty eating, intravenous fluids may be needed to rehydrate you. - Hospitalization: If your symptoms are severe or you have a weakened immune system, you may need to be hospitalized for treatment. It is important to rest and drink plenty of fluids to help your body recover from pneumonia. Follow your doctor's instructions for any prescribed medications and ensure you complete the full course of antibiotics if they are prescribed.

Conclusion

Pneumonia is a serious respiratory infection that requires medical attention. Symptoms can worsen quickly, especially in high-risk individuals, so it is important to see a doctor if you experience any symptoms. Treatment depends on the cause of the infection and may include antibiotics, rest, and intravenous fluids.

Chapter 22: Tuberculosis: Signs and Symptoms

Tuberculosis, often called TB, is a bacterial infection that spreads through the air. TB primarily affects the lungs, but can also infect other parts of the body, such as the kidneys, spine, and brain. It is a serious respiratory condition that requires prompt medical attention. In this chapter, we will discuss the signs and symptoms of tuberculosis.

EARLY SIGNS AND SYMPTOMS

In most cases, the early signs and symptoms of TB are mild and non-specific. They often include:

Chronic Cough

The most common symptom of TB is a persistent cough that lasts for three or more weeks. This cough may be accompanied by mucus or blood.

Fever

Fever is another common symptom of TB. The body temperature may rise above 100.4 F (38 C) in the afternoon or evening.

Night Sweats

Sweating at night, even if it's cold, is a typical symptom of tuberculosis. Wetting the bedclothes, sheets, and pajamas.

Unexplained Weight Loss

Tuberculosis can cause significant weight loss. If you are losing weight unintentionally, it would be best to seek medical attention.

ADVANCED SIGNS AND SYMPTOMS

If tuberculosis is not treated promptly, the symptoms can become more severe and may include:

Chest Pain

Severe chest pain while breathing or coughing can be a symptom of tuberculosis. This is typically worse in the morning.

Shortness of Breath

Tuberculosis can cause shortness of breath and difficulty breathing. This can be especially noticeable during physical activity.

Wheezing

Wheezing and whistling sounds when breathing can also be a symptom of tuberculosis.

Coughing Up Blood

In advanced stages of tuberculosis, coughing up blood or hemoptysis can occur.

Fatigue

Experiencing persistent fatigue and lack of energy could be a symptom of tuberculosis.

CONCLUSION

Tuberculosis is a severe respiratory condition that requires urgent medical attention. If you experience any of the symptoms mentioned above, seek medical attention immediately. Remember, early detection and treatment of tuberculosis can help prevent the spread of the illness and improve your chances of recovery.

Chapter 23: Lung Cancer: Signs, Symptoms, and Diagnosis

Lung cancer is a serious and potentially fatal condition that affects many people worldwide. It is the second most common cancer in men and women and is responsible for a large number of deaths every year.

TYPES OF LUNG CANCER

There are two main types of lung cancer: small cell lung cancer (SCLC) and non-small cell lung cancer (NSCLC). SCLC tends to spread more quickly than NSCLC and is usually associated with smoking. NSCLC is more common and develops more slowly than SCLC.

SIGNS AND SYMPTOMS OF LUNG CANCER

The symptoms of lung cancer can vary depending on where the cancer is located in the lung and how far it has spread. Common symptoms include:

1. Persistent cough

A cough that doesn't go away or gets worse over time is one of the most common symptoms of lung cancer.

2. Shortness of breath

Difficulty breathing or shortness of breath can be caused by lung cancer blocking or narrowing the airway.

3. Chest pain

Persistent chest pain that worsens when coughing or breathing deeply is a symptom of lung cancer.

4. Unexplained weight loss

Lung cancer can cause a loss of appetite and subsequent weight loss.

5. Fatigue

Feeling excessively tired or weak can be an indication of lung cancer.

6. Hoarseness

Hoarseness or other changes in the voice may result from lung cancer pressing on a nerve.

7. Coughing up blood

Coughing up blood or rust-colored sputum can be a sign of lung cancer.

DIAGNOSIS OF LUNG CANCER

Lung cancer is typically diagnosed through a combination of tests and examinations. These can include a chest X-ray, CT scans, PET scans, and biopsies. The goal is to identify whether or not a tumor is present, and if so, determine its size, location, and if it has begun to spread. It is important to seek medical attention if you experience any of the symptoms associated with lung cancer. The earlier the cancer is detected and treated, the greater the chance of successful treatment.

Chapter 24: Finding Support for Respiratory Conditions

Living with a respiratory condition like COPD or any other related disease can be a challenging experience. In many cases, patients feel isolated and misunderstood, which can increase anxiety and depression. However, finding the right kind of support can make a significant difference in managing the disease and improving the quality of life.

SUPPORT GROUPS

One of the most helpful resources for people living with respiratory conditions is support groups. Support groups provide a safe space for people with similar challenges to share their experiences, ask questions, and offer encouragement. Many support groups meet in person, but there are also online support groups that can be helpful, especially for people who are unable to attend in-person meetings due to physical limitations.

Finding a support group

There are many ways to find a support group in your area. Hospitals, community centers, and religious organizations often host support group meetings. Your doctor or nurse can also refer you to local support groups. You can also search for online support groups through websites like Facebook or Meetup.

COUNSELING

Counseling can also be beneficial for people living with respiratory conditions. Counseling can help individuals manage symptoms that often accompany respiratory conditions such as anxiety, depression, and stress. Counseling can also help patients improve communication with their healthcare providers, which can lead to better disease management.

Types of counseling

There are different types of counseling that can be helpful for people with respiratory conditions. One form of counseling that is commonly used is cognitive-behavioral therapy (CBT). CBT focuses on changing negative thought patterns to improve well-being. Other forms of counseling, such as talk therapy or group therapy, can also be beneficial.

FINANCIAL ASSISTANCE

Living with a respiratory condition can be expensive, and many people struggle to pay for their treatments and medications. However, there are resources available to help offset the cost of care.

Government assistance

Many government programs can provide financial assistance to people living with respiratory conditions. Medicare and Medicaid, for example, can help cover the costs of treatment and medication. Veterans can also receive financial assistance through the Department of Veterans Affairs.

Non-profit organizations

There are also non-profit organizations that can provide financial assistance to people living with respiratory conditions. The American Lung Association, for example, offers financial assistance for medication costs. Other organizations offer grants or other financial support to individuals who need help paying for care.

CONCLUSION

Living with a respiratory condition can be challenging, but finding the right support can make a significant difference. Support groups, counseling, and financial assistance are just a few of the resources available to help manage the disease. By seeking out these resources, individuals can improve their quality of life and better manage their respiratory condition.

Chapter 25: Navigating the Health Care System

Living with chronic obstructive pulmonary disease (COPD) and other respiratory conditions can be challenging and may require frequent medical attention. Navigating the health care system can be overwhelming, but it is essential to understand how to access the care you need. In this chapter, we will discuss some tips for navigating the health care system when living with COPD or other respiratory conditions.

UNDERSTANDING YOUR HEALTH INSURANCE

One of the first steps in navigating the health care system is understanding your health insurance. If you have health insurance, it is important to understand what services are covered and what your out-of-pocket costs may be. Be sure to review your plan's benefits and limitations, as well as any deductibles, copays, or coinsurance amounts. If you are eligible for Medicare, you may be able to receive coverage for a variety of services related to your respiratory condition. Medicare may cover services such as pulmonary rehabilitation, oxygen therapy, and certain medications. It is important to understand the specific services that are covered under your plan and any associated costs.

FINDING THE RIGHT HEALTH CARE PROVIDERS

When living with COPD or other respiratory conditions, it is important to find a health care provider who can help manage your condition. This may include a primary care physician, pulmonologist, respiratory therapist, or other specialist. To find the right health care providers, start by asking for referrals from your current provider or friends and family. You can also search online for providers in your area who specialize in treating respiratory conditions.

PREPARING FOR APPOINTMENTS

Preparing for appointments with your health care provider can help ensure that you get the most out of your visits. Before your appointment, make a list of any symptoms or concerns you have. Be sure to bring a list of any medications you are taking, as well as any recent test results or medical records. During your appointment, be sure to ask any questions you have and share any concerns you may have about your condition. Your health care provider can work with you to develop a personalized treatment plan and help you manage your symptoms.

ADVOCATING FOR YOUR HEALTH

Advocating for your health is an important part of managing your condition. This may include speaking up about your symptoms or concerns, asking for additional tests or referrals, and ensuring that you receive the care you need. If you feel that your concerns are not being addressed or that you are not receiving the care you need, don't be afraid to speak up. Consider seeking a second opinion or talking to a patient advocate for support.

CONCLUSION

Navigating the health care system can be challenging, but it is essential to understand how to access the care you need when living with COPD or other respiratory conditions. By understanding your health insurance, finding the right health care providers, preparing for appointments, and advocating for your health, you can ensure that you receive the care you need to manage your condition.

Chapter 26: Financial Assistance for COPD and Respiratory Conditions

COPD and other respiratory conditions can come with a high cost of treatment, and for those who are uninsured or underinsured, the financial burden can be overwhelming. Fortunately, there are several options available for financial assistance.

MEDICARE COVERAGE

For those over the age of 65, Medicare provides coverage for COPD and respiratory treatments, including oxygen therapy and certain medications. It is important to research the specific coverage options provided by Medicare and to enroll in the appropriate plan.

MEDICAID COVERAGE

Medicaid provides coverage for low-income individuals and families, including those with COPD and other respiratory conditions. Coverage includes doctor visits, hospital stays, and necessary medications. Qualifications for Medicaid vary by state, so it is important to research the options available in your area.

PRESCRIPTION DRUG ASSISTANCE PROGRAMS

Many pharmaceutical companies offer patient assistance programs for those who cannot afford their medications. These programs provide discounts or free medications to eligible individuals. It is important to research the specific programs offered by the medication's manufacturer and to apply for assistance.

PATIENT ASSISTANCE CHARITIES

There are several charitable organizations that provide financial assistance for COPD and respiratory treatments. These organizations include the American Lung Association and the COPD Foundation. Their programs offer financial assistance for medications, oxygen therapy, and other treatment costs.

CROWDFUNDING

Crowdfunding websites provide an opportunity for individuals to raise funds for medical treatments and expenses. These websites allow individuals to create a campaign and share their story and financial need with others. It is important to research and carefully consider the terms and conditions of each crowdfunding website, as they may have fees and regulations.

COPD and other respiratory conditions can be financially burdensome, but there are options available for financial assistance. It is important to research the options provided by Medicare and Medicaid, as well as patient assistance programs and charitable organizations. Crowdfunding can also be a viable option for those with significant financial need. No one should have to choose between their health and their financial well-being, and with the help of these resources, individuals with respiratory conditions can access the care they need.

Chapter 27: Advocacy for Respiratory Health

One of the biggest challenges for individuals living with respiratory conditions is the lack of awareness and advocacy for respiratory health. Many individuals with respiratory conditions have difficulty accessing proper healthcare and treatment options. This is why advocacy for respiratory health is so important. Advocacy for respiratory health can take many forms. It involves efforts to increase public awareness and education about respiratory conditions, as well as advocacy for policy and legislative changes that improve access to healthcare and treatment for individuals living with respiratory conditions. One way to advocate for respiratory health is to get involved in a local or national respiratory health organization. These organizations often provide resources and support for individuals living with respiratory conditions and their families, as well as advocacy efforts aimed at improving respiratory health policy and legislation. Another way to advocate for respiratory health is to participate in respiratory health events and campaigns. This can include participating in respiratory health walks or runs, wearing respiratory health awareness ribbons or shirts, or sharing information about respiratory conditions on social media or other platforms. In addition to individual advocacy efforts, it is important to support and fund research into respiratory health. Research into respiratory conditions can help improve diagnosis and treatment options, as well as increase public awareness and understanding of respiratory conditions. Advocacy for respiratory health is essential for improving the lives of individuals living with respiratory conditions and reducing morbidity and mortality rates associated with these conditions. It is important for individuals, healthcare professionals, and policymakers to work together to improve respiratory health outcomes and ensure that everyone has access to quality respiratory healthcare.

Conclusion

Advocacy for respiratory health is crucial for improving respiratory health outcomes and reducing morbidity and mortality rates associated with respiratory conditions. It involves efforts to increase public awareness and education about respiratory conditions, as well as advocacy for policy and legislative changes that improve access to healthcare and treatment for individuals living with respiratory conditions. By working together, individuals, healthcare professionals, and policymakers can improve respiratory health outcomes and ensure that everyone has access to quality respiratory healthcare.

Chapter 28: Research on COPD and Respiratory Conditions

Chronic obstructive pulmonary disease (COPD) and other respiratory conditions are serious illnesses that affect millions of people worldwide. Given the widespread prevalence of these conditions, researchers have been studying them extensively in order to develop better treatments and improve patient outcomes.

CURRENT RESEARCH ON COPD

Numerous studies are currently being conducted on COPD and related respiratory conditions. One area of research is focused on identifying the best ways to manage COPD symptoms, reduce exacerbations, and improve quality of life for patients with the condition. Researchers are also working to develop new medications and treatment options that can help to slow the progression of the disease.

Another area of research is focused on identifying risk factors for COPD and developing strategies to prevent the disease from developing in the first place. Smoking is a well-known risk factor for COPD, but researchers are also exploring other potential causes, such as air pollution, workplace exposures, and genetics.

PROGRESS IN RESPIRATORY RESEARCH

Thanks to ongoing research efforts, significant progress has been made in the treatment of COPD and other respiratory conditions. For example, the development of new medications (such as bronchodilators and inhaled steroids) and treatment approaches (such as pulmonary rehabilitation and oxygen therapy) have resulted in better symptom management and improved quality of life for many patients.

In addition to developing new treatments, researchers are also exploring new strategies for diagnosing and monitoring respiratory conditions. For example, new imaging technologies (such as computed tomography and magnetic resonance imaging) have allowed for more accurate diagnosis of early stage lung cancer and other respiratory conditions.

FUTURE DIRECTIONS IN RESPIRATORY RESEARCH

Despite progress in the treatment and management of respiratory conditions, there is still much work to be done. Future directions in respiratory research include identifying new risk factors for respiratory illnesses, improving early detection and diagnosis, developing more personalized treatment approaches, and identifying ways to prevent the development and progression of respiratory conditions.

In addition, researchers are exploring the potential of regenerative medicine and stem cell therapies for repairing damaged lung tissue and improving respiratory function in patients with COPD and other respiratory conditions.

THE IMPORTANCE OF SUPPORTING RESPIRATORY RESEARCH

Given the significant impact of respiratory conditions on individuals and society as a whole, it is critical that we continue to support research efforts in this area. Funding for respiratory research can help to accelerate progress in developing new treatments, improving patient outcomes, and ultimately reducing the burden of respiratory illnesses on patients and their families.

By investing in research on COPD and other respiratory conditions, we can help to ensure that individuals with these conditions have access to the best possible care and treatment options. With ongoing research and advances in medical technology, we can make a meaningful difference in the lives of those affected by respiratory illnesses.

Chapter 29: The Future of COPD Treatment

Chronic Obstructive Pulmonary Disease, or COPD, is a chronic respiratory disease that affects millions of people around the world. At present, there is no cure for COPD, and current treatments only aim to manage symptoms and slow down the progression of the disease. However, there is ongoing research into new and innovative treatments that could change the landscape of COPD treatment in the future.

NEW DRUG THERAPIES

One of the most promising areas of research for COPD is the development of new drug therapies. At present, the most commonly used medications for COPD are bronchodilators and corticosteroids. While these medications can be effective at managing symptoms, they do not address the underlying cause of the disease.

Researchers are looking at new drug therapies that target inflammation and repair damage to the lungs. One potential drug is called GLPG1690, which is designed to reduce inflammation in the lungs. Another drug in development is called Verona Pharma's RPL554, which is designed to widen the airways. Clinical trials have shown promising results for both these drugs, and they could be available within the next few years.

STEM CELL THERAPY

Stem cell therapy is a relatively new approach to treating COPD that involves using stem cells to repair damaged lung tissue. The idea is that stem cells can differentiate into lung tissue and replace damaged cells, thus improving lung function. Several studies have shown that stem cell therapy can improve lung function in people with COPD. However, more research is needed to determine the safety and efficacy of this therapy. Researchers are also exploring different types of stem cells and different delivery methods to improve the results of this treatment.

LUNG VOLUME REDUCTION SURGERY

Lung volume reduction surgery is a surgical procedure that involves removing damaged tissue from the lungs. The idea is that by removing damaged tissue, the remaining healthy tissue can function more efficiently and improve lung function. While lung volume reduction surgery has been around for several decades, it has traditionally been a high-risk procedure with significant side effects. However, new advances in surgical techniques, as well as better patient selection and management, have made this treatment option safer and more effective.

THE ROLE OF PRECISION MEDICINE

Precision medicine is an approach to healthcare that involves tailoring treatments to individual patients based on their genetic makeup, environment, and lifestyle factors. This approach could be particularly valuable for people with COPD, as the disease is influenced by a variety of factors. For example, researchers are looking at genetic biomarkers that could help identify people at risk of developing COPD or predict disease progression. This information could be used to develop targeted treatments that address the specific underlying mechanisms of the disease.

CONCLUSION

While there is currently no cure for COPD, there is ongoing research into new and innovative treatments that could change that in the future. From new drug therapies to stem cell treatments to precision medicine, the future of COPD treatment is promising. As research continues, there is hope that we can improve the lives of millions of people living with this chronic respiratory disease.